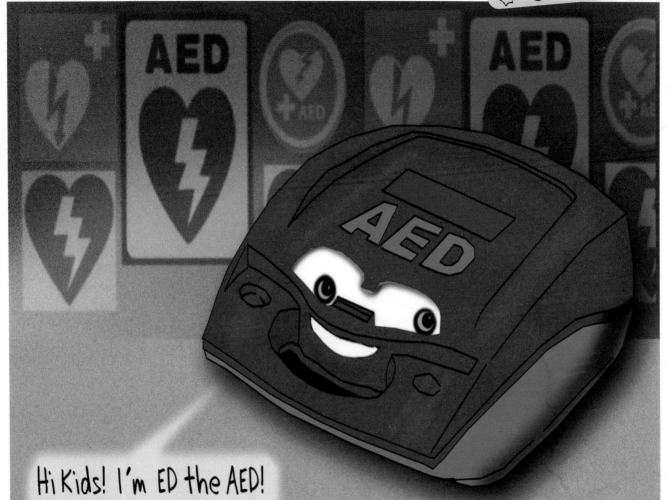

Hi Kids! I'm ED the AED!

AED stands for Automated External Defibrilalltor. Sound it out with me...

"aw toe may ted - eck stur nall - de fib rill a tor".

I know these are BIG words but I have a BIG and EXCITING job!

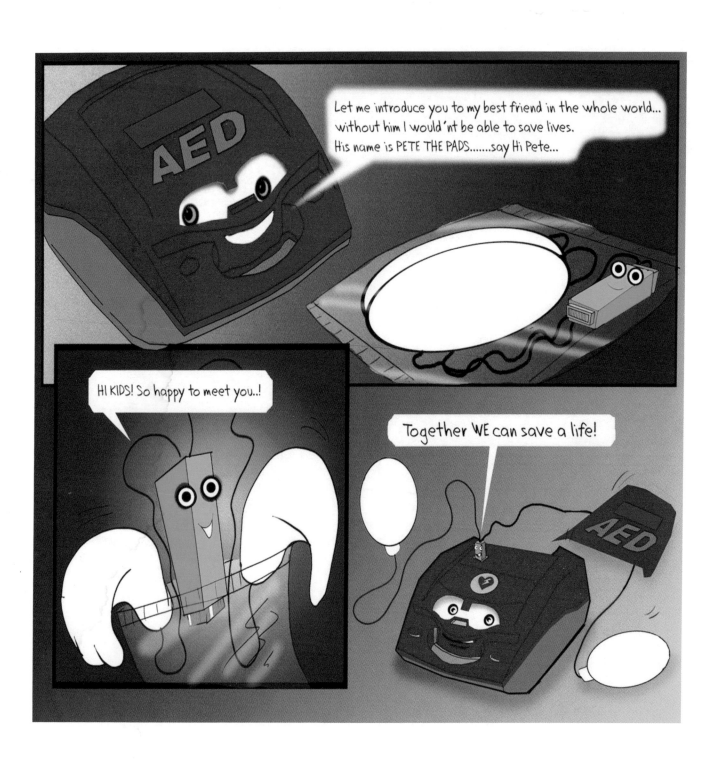

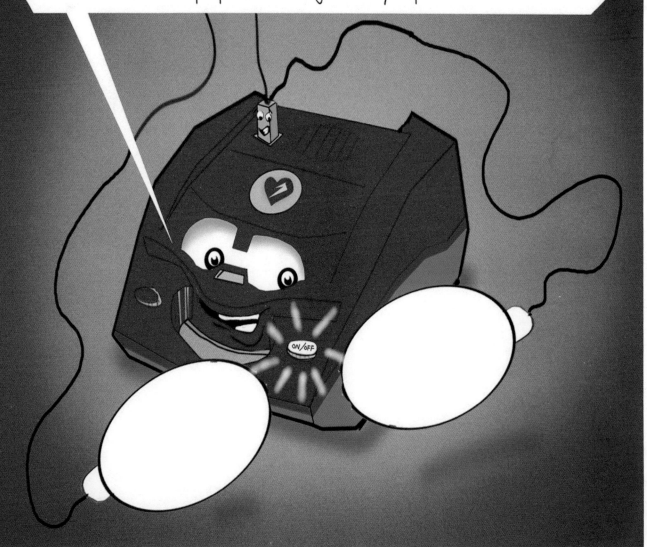

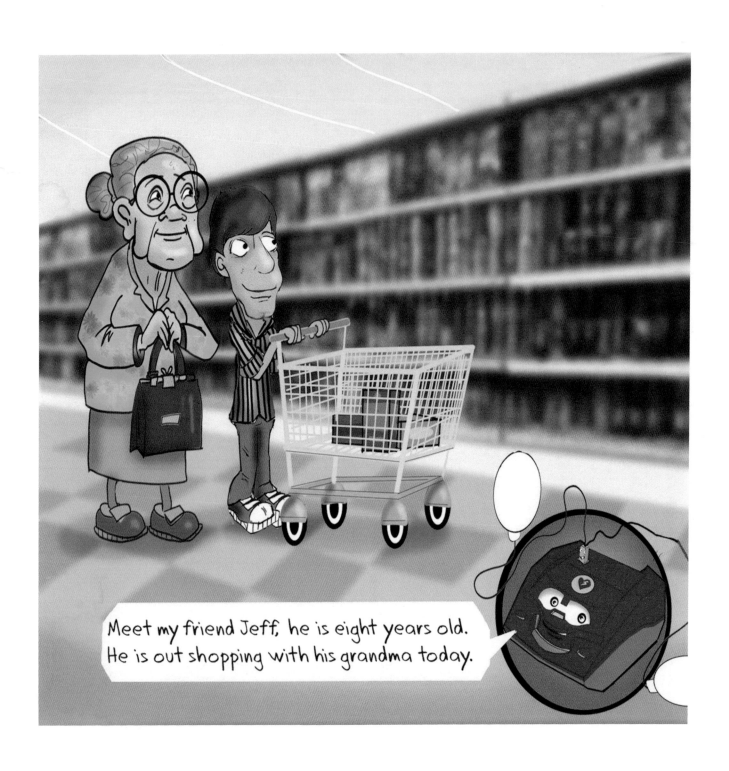

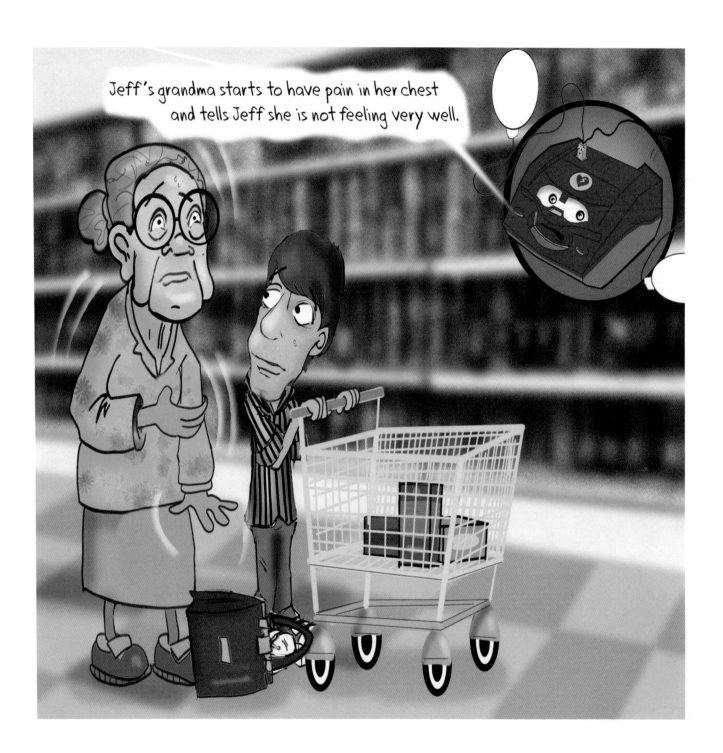

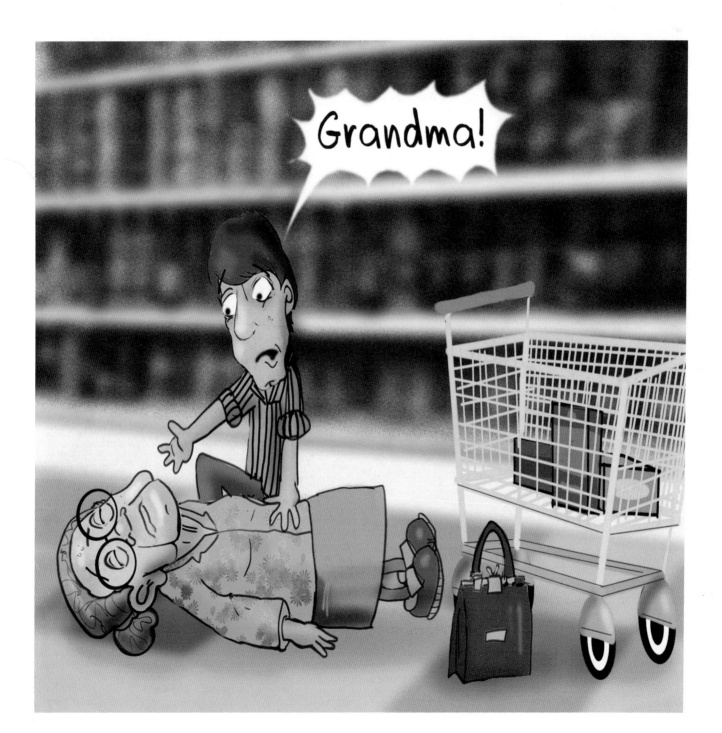

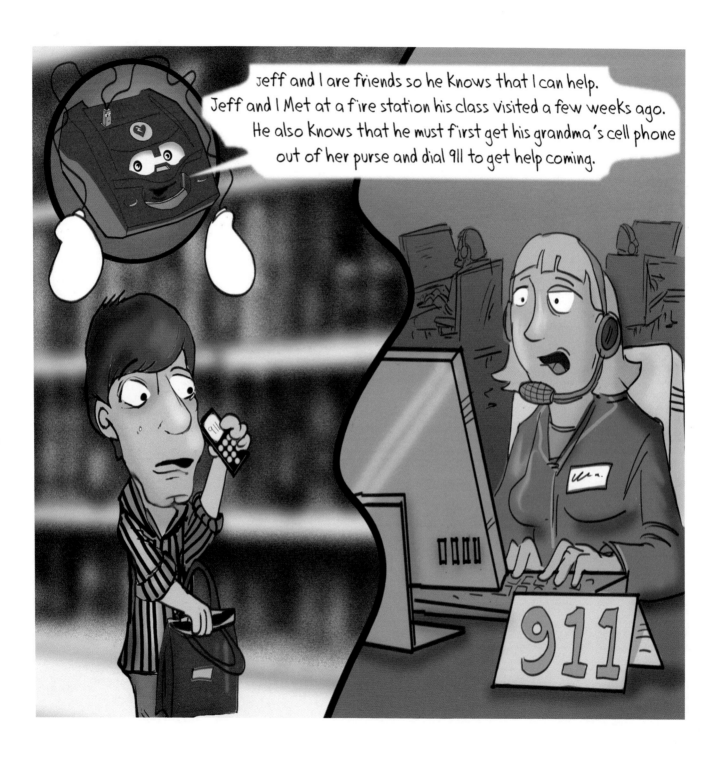

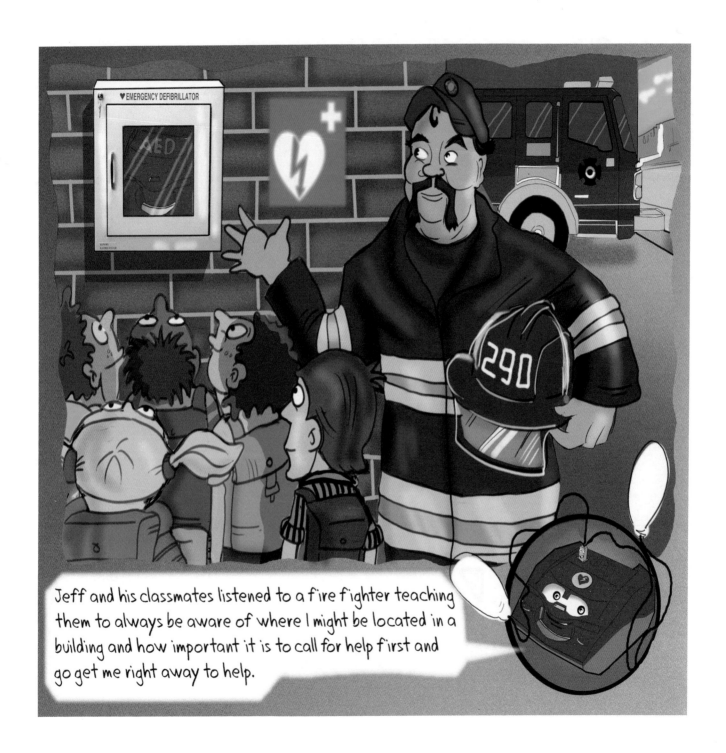

Jeff and his classmates listened to a fire fighter teaching them to always be aware of where I might be located in a building and how important it is to call for help first and go get me right away to help.

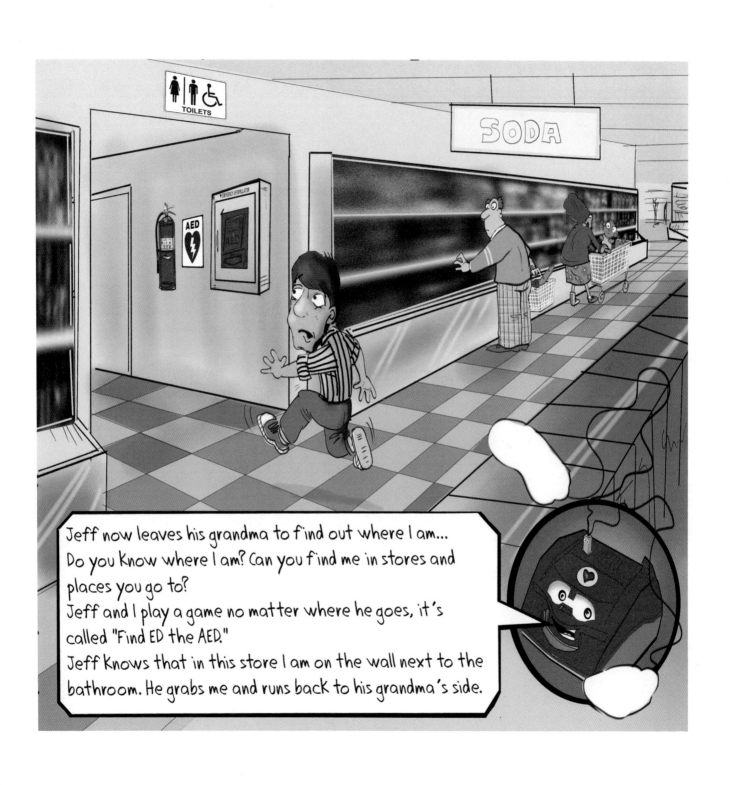

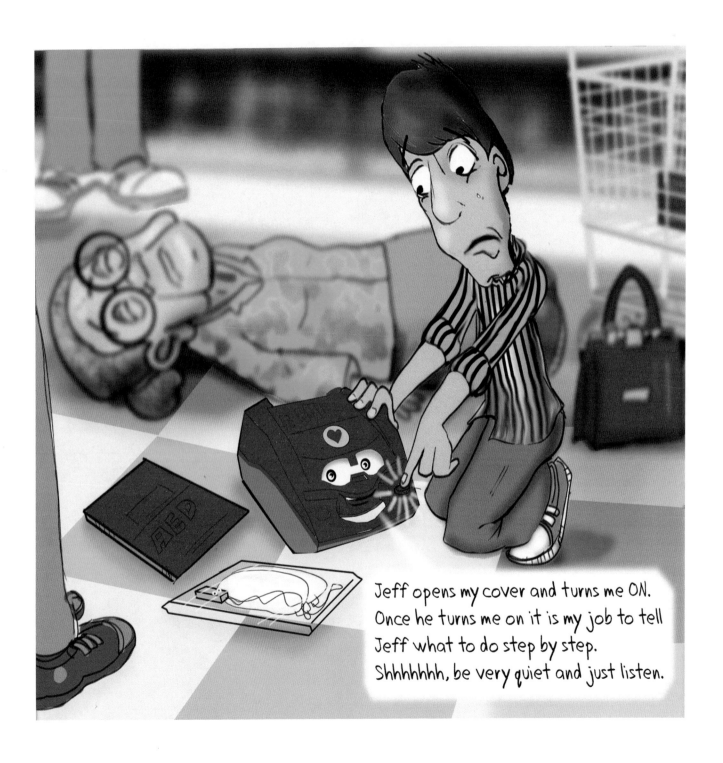

Jeff opens my cover and turns me ON.
Once he turns me on it is my job to tell
Jeff what to do step by step.
Shhhhhhh, be very quiet and just listen.

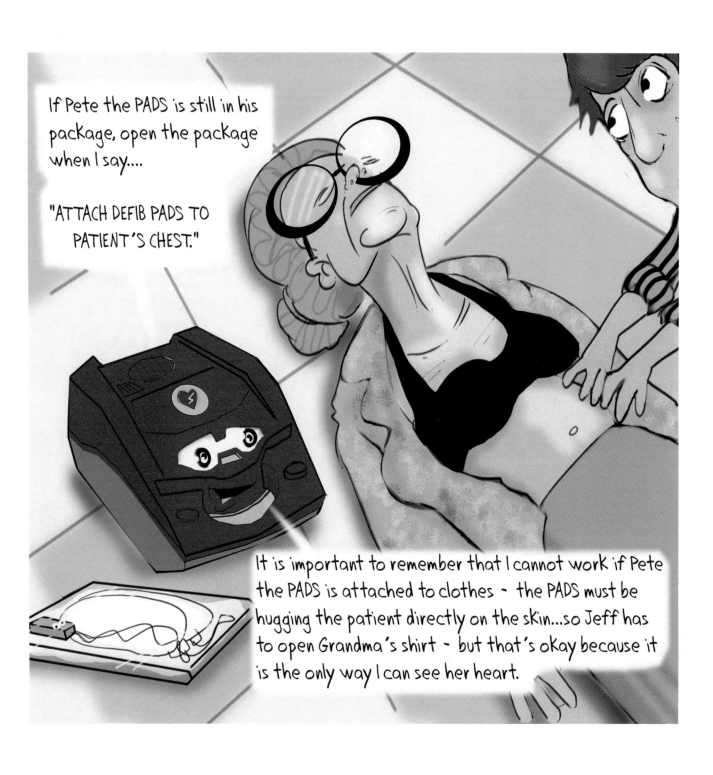

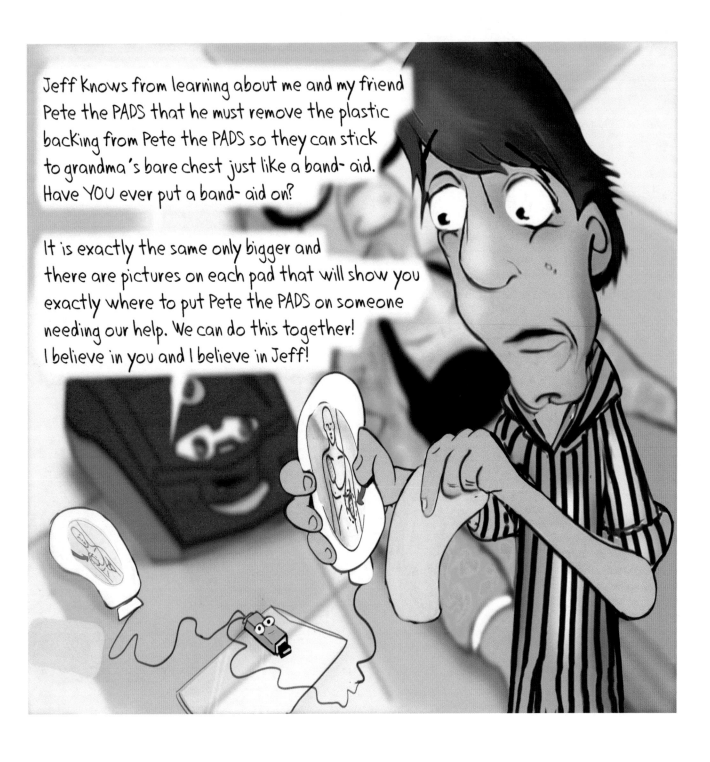

Jeff knows from learning about me and my friend Pete the PADS that he must remove the plastic backing from Pete the PADS so they can stick to grandma's bare chest just like a band-aid. Have YOU ever put a band-aid on?

It is exactly the same only bigger and there are pictures on each pad that will show you exactly where to put Pete the PADS on someone needing our help. We can do this together! I believe in you and I believe in Jeff!

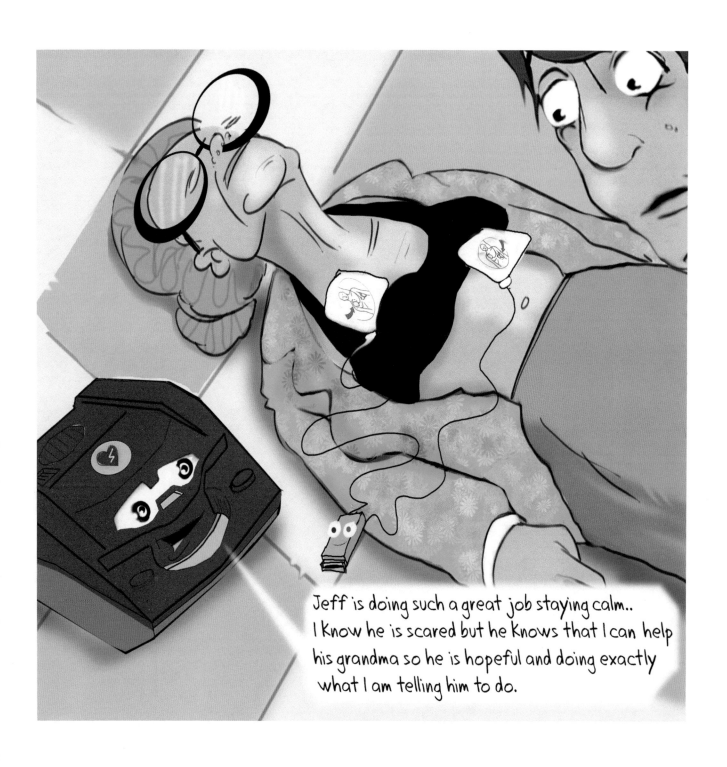

Jeff is doing such a great job staying calm..
I know he is scared but he knows that I can help
his grandma so he is hopeful and doing exactly
what I am telling him to do.

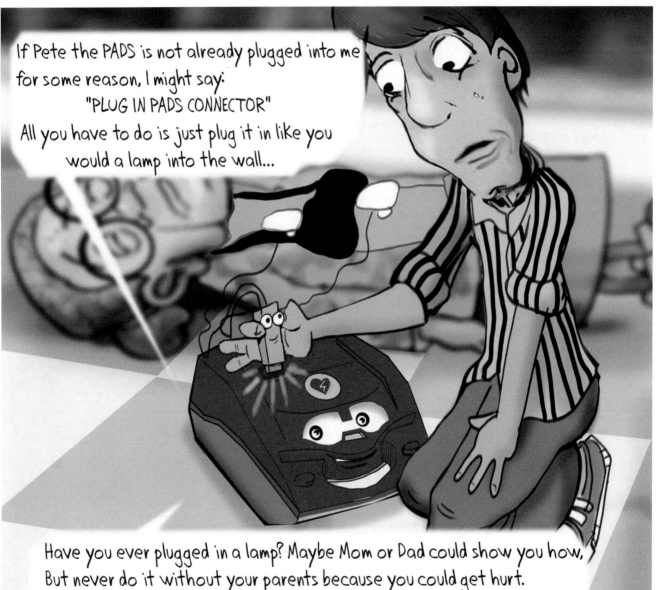

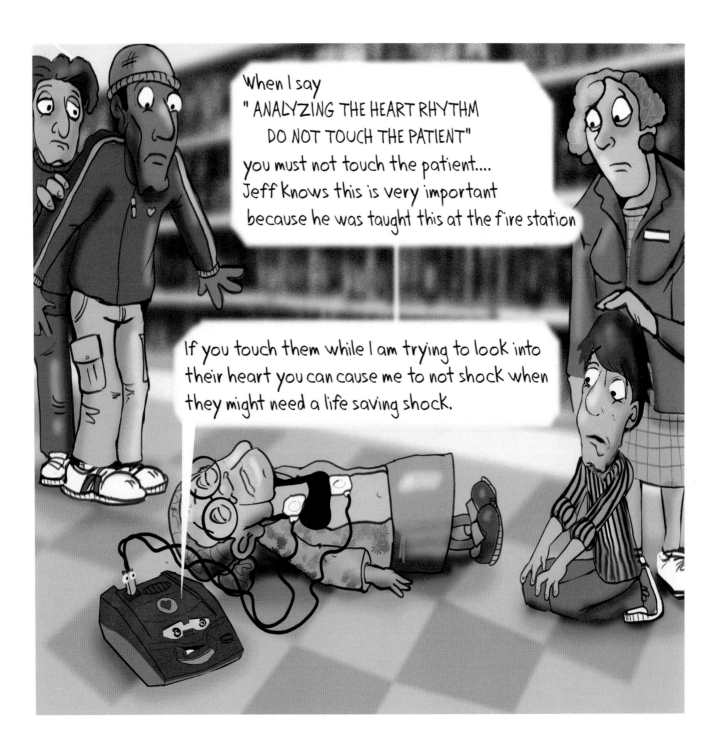

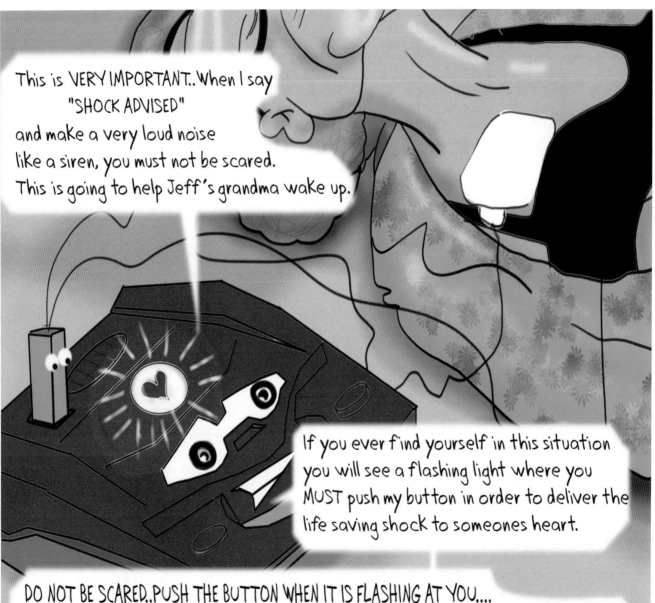

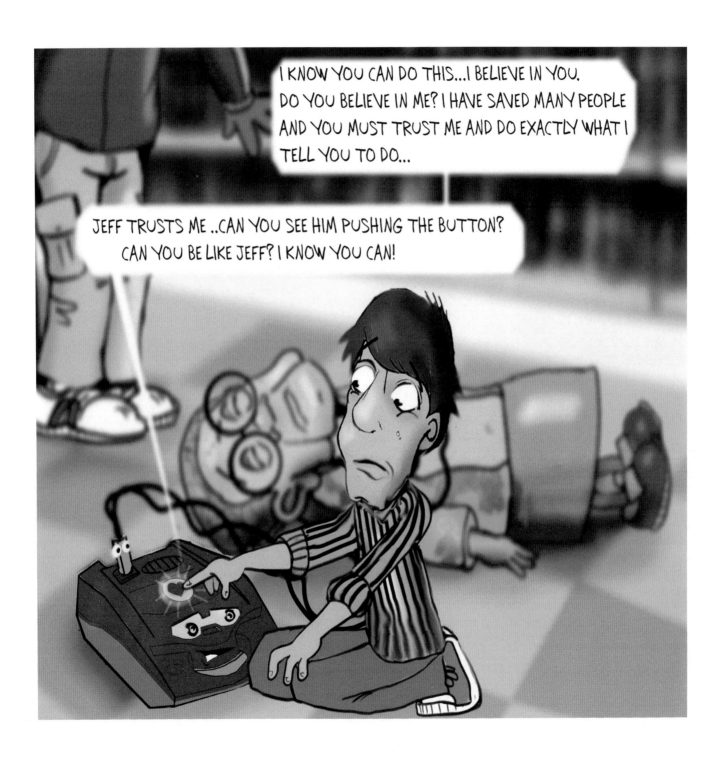

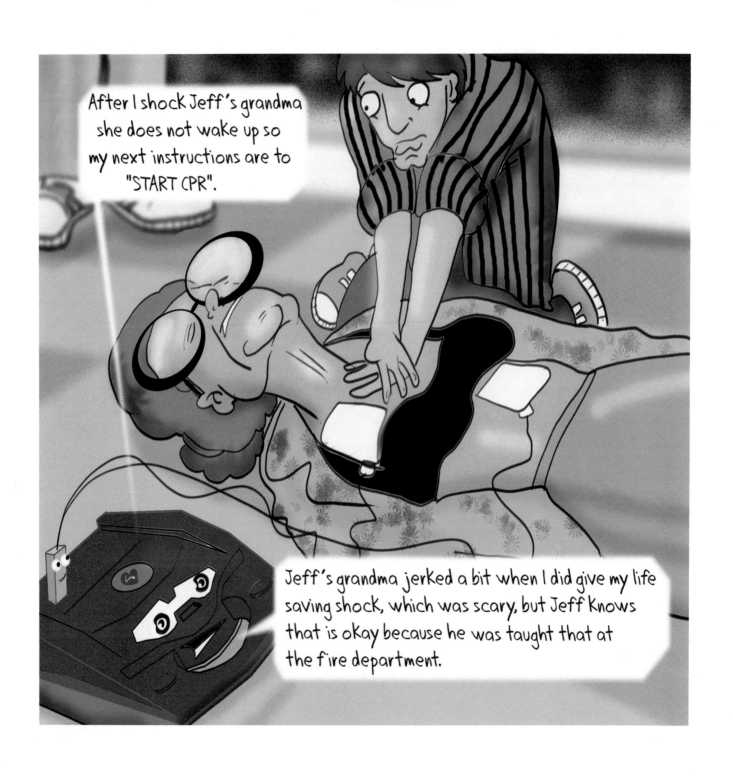

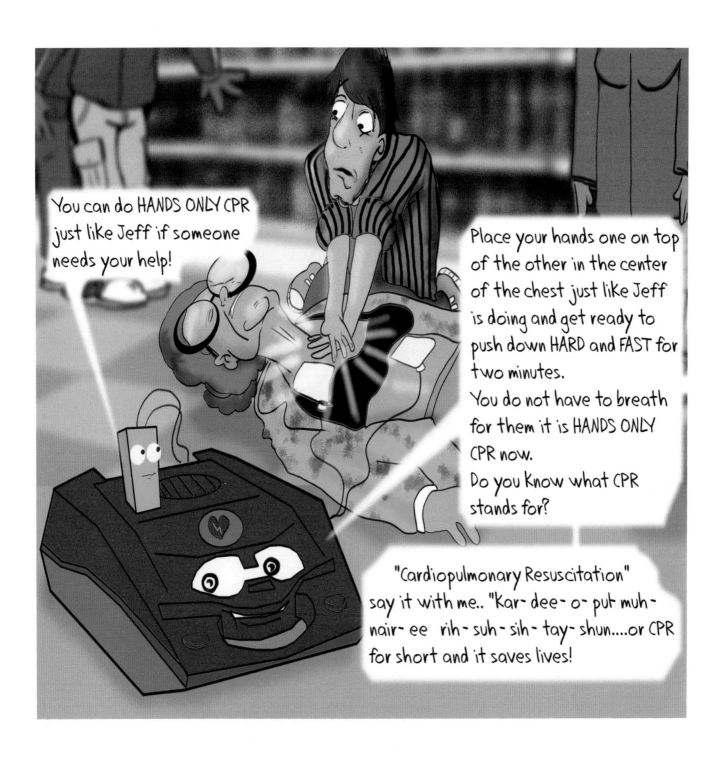

Cardio means "of the heart" and pulmonary means "of the lungs" and resuscitation is a medical word that means "to revive" or to bring back to life which is where I come in because only AED's can bring someone back to life in the right situation. CPR is a very important thing to do though because it buys valuable time until I (the AED) can be brought to the patient's side and CPR saves the brain from dying.

When the heart stops pumping on its own then no oxygen is going to the brain and the brain will die very quickly. CPR keeps the brain from dying but I am the only thing that can correct what is wrong with the heart and help the person to have blood flow and breathing again on their own.

When the heart stops pumping it is quivering like a bowl of shaking Jell-O the only thing that can stop the jiggling which does not produce blood flow is MY electricity! Once the heart is stopped with my electricity it can re-start itself and then pump correctly again!

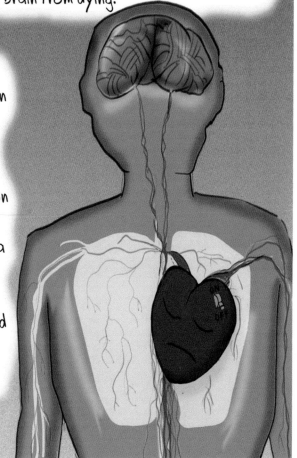

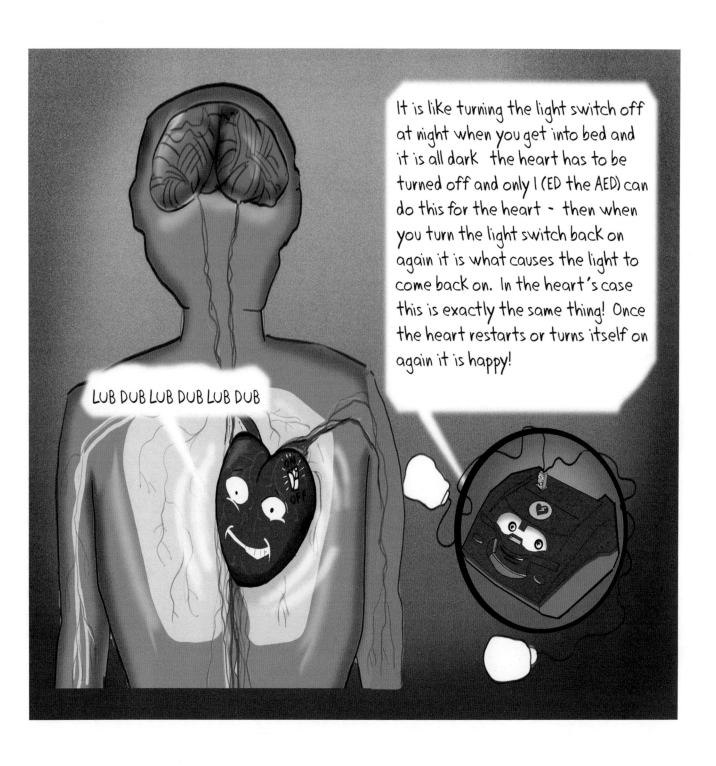

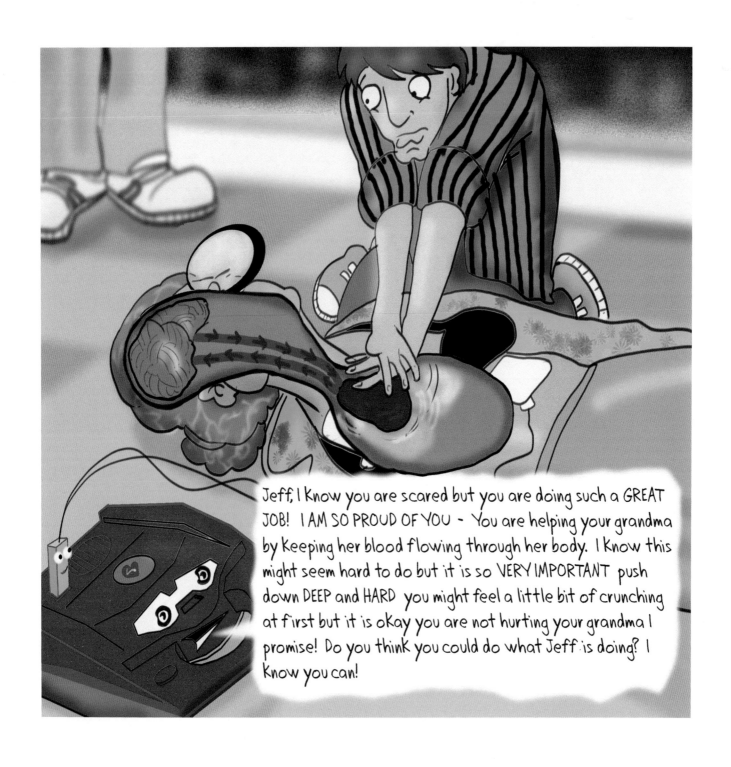

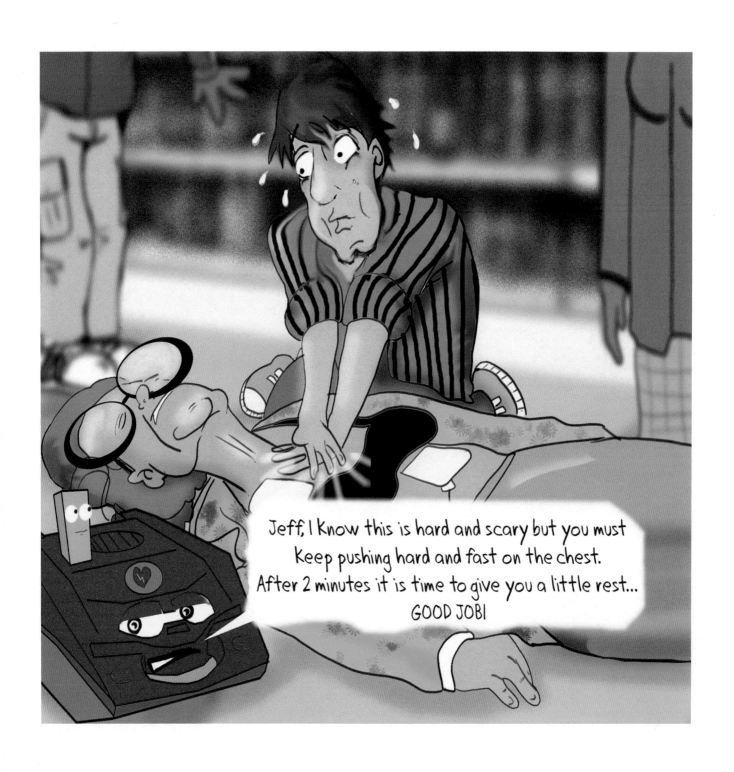

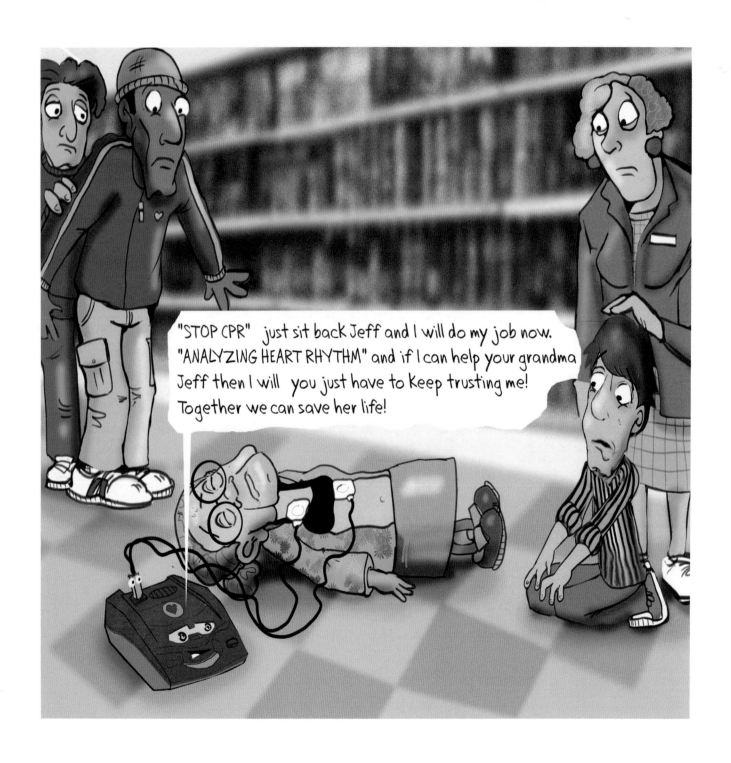

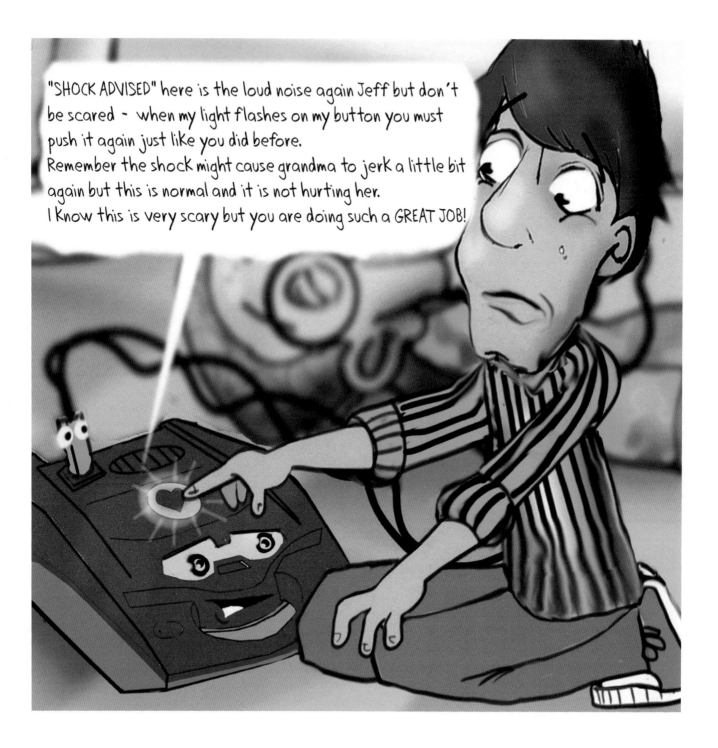

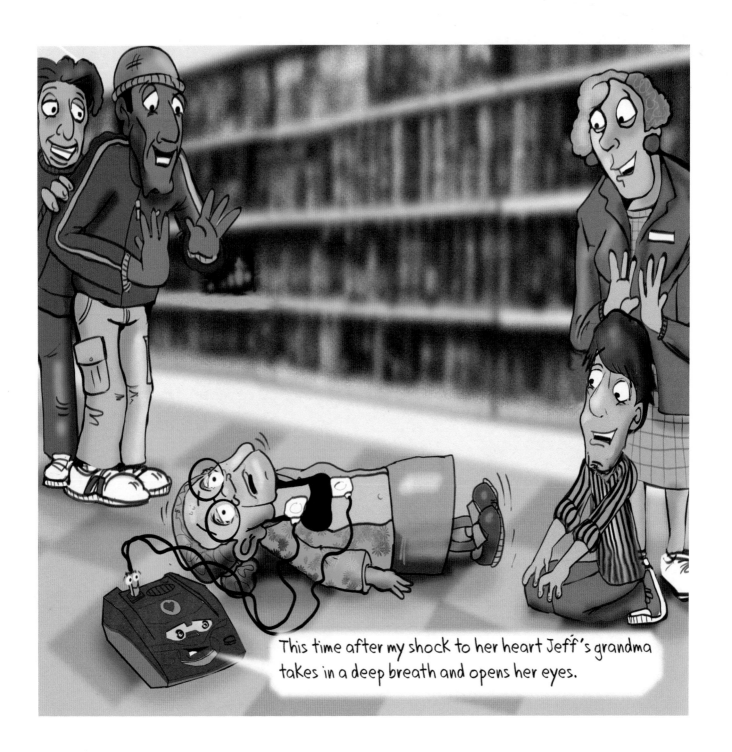

This time after my shock to her heart Jeff's grandma takes in a deep breath and opens her eyes.

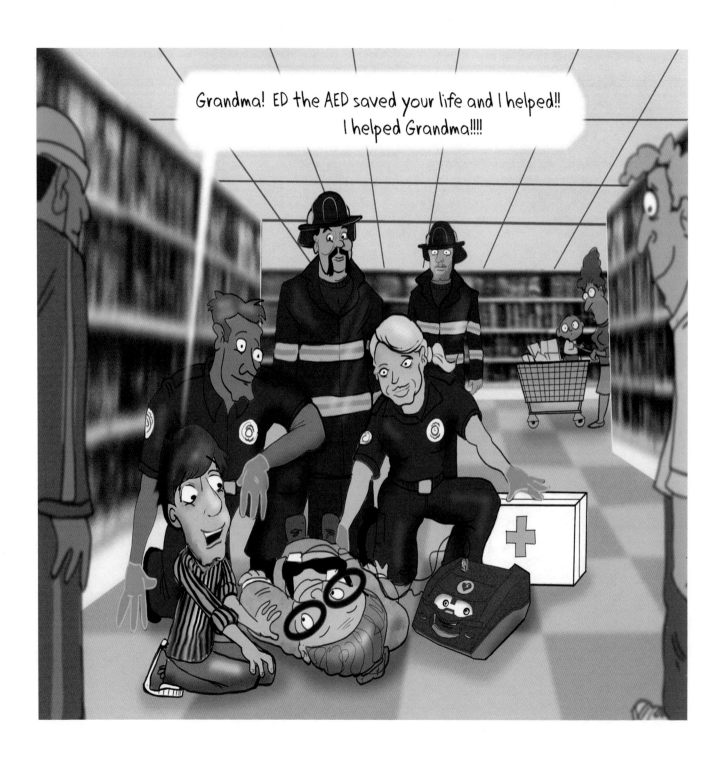

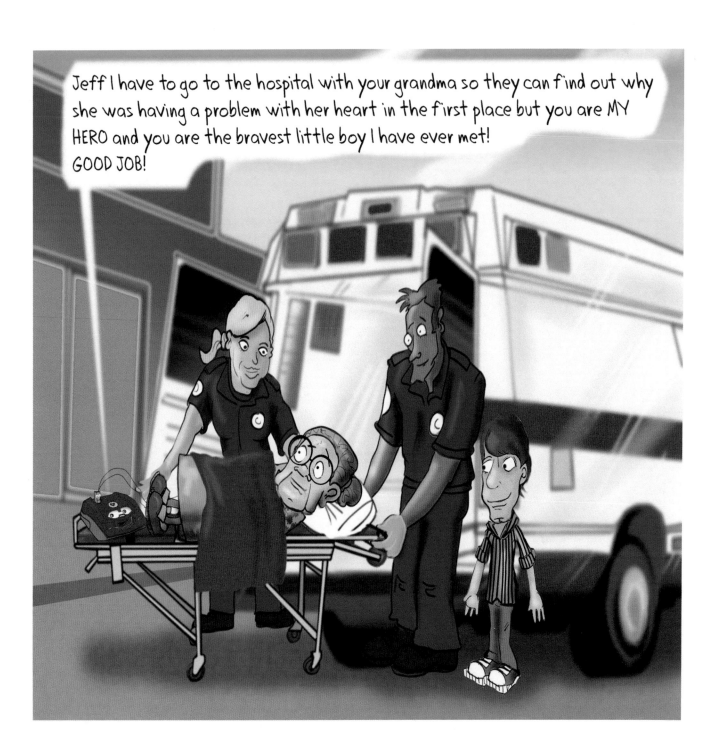

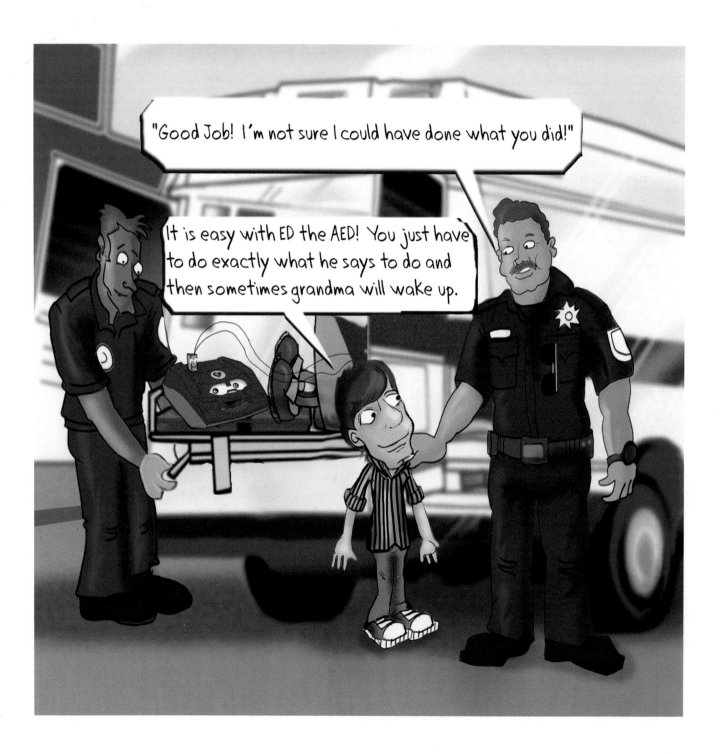

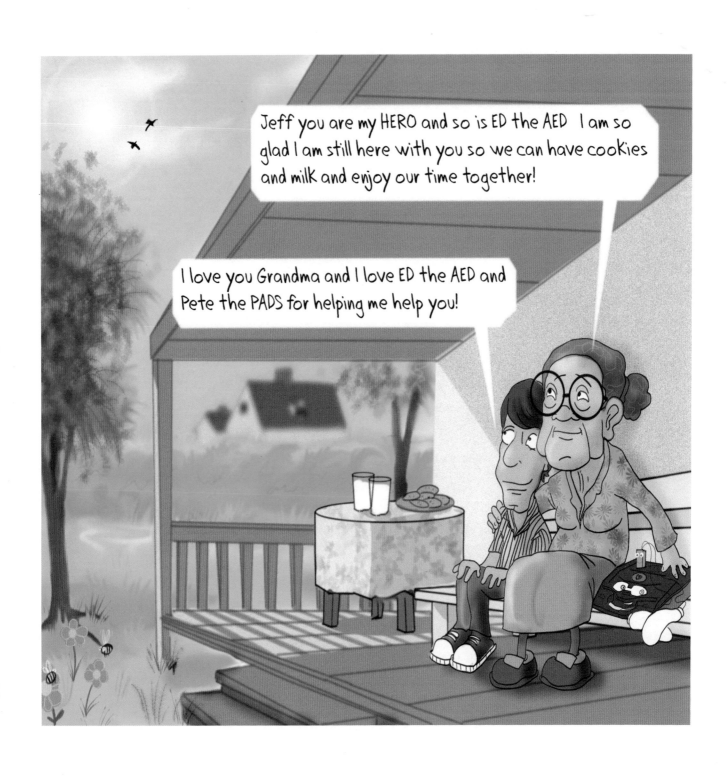

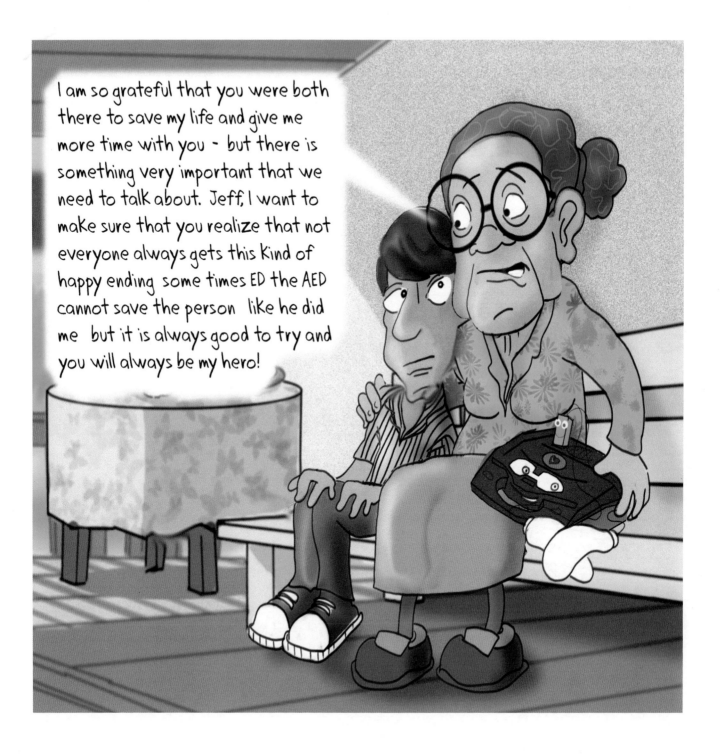

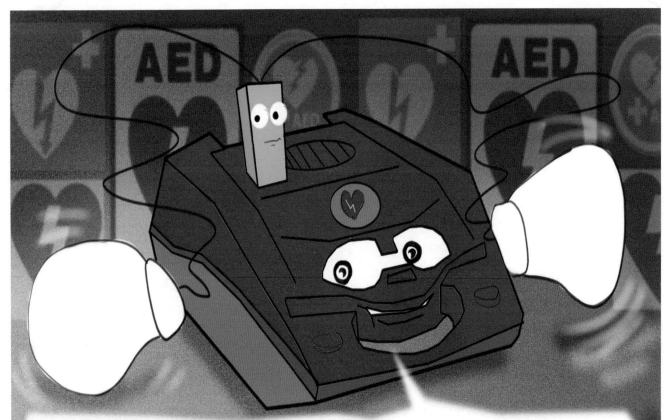

Do YOU believe that you are a HERO even if you cannot save the person you are helping? You must believe this because not everyone can be saved. Some people have heart problems that are too hard to fix. This is NOT your fault. If you help then you are a HERO every single time no matter what the outcome.

You must remember that some times people die and we do not understand why - but it is always good to try because I can help people in the right situations. It is always good to act quickly and do what you can to help. Just remember to TURN ME ON FIRST and then do exactly as I say   you are a HERO for trying no matter what the outcome!

Made in the USA
Charleston, SC
01 March 2014